Leak

MW01170158

Why A Leaky Gut May Be The Root Of All Your Health Problems And How To Cure It With Natural Home Remedies

(Including A 4 Weeks Meal Plan To Detox And Improve Digestive Health)

Eileen Dumont

Introduction

From the name, you might think that it only affects the digestive system but leaky gut syndrome may be the cause of a wide range of serious chronic diseases that affect us today. According to medical researches, the leaky gut syndrome could be the cause of your food allergies, thyroid disease, slow metabolism, and autoimmune conditions. In addition, over time, more and more people are suffering from this condition.

This book will be a guide to healing the leaky gut syndrome and a breakthrough to the health problems that you have been struggling with, because of leaky gut syndrome.

Table of Contents

An Understanding Of Leaky Gut Syndrome

A thin semi-permeable lining protects our digestive tract. Think of it this way. Imagine your digestive tract lining to be like a sieve with extremely tiny holes that is very selective with what goes through and what does not enter the bloodstream. The gut lining in our intestines works as a barrier that keeps out bigger particles not important for our system while allowing the absorption of vitamins and minerals from the food we eat. In reality, the sieve is a mucin layer.

Often referred to as increased intestinal permeability, a leaky gut occurs when the 'sieve' in our digestive system gets damaged with the development of bigger holes. This ends up allowing bigger particles to enter the bloodstream with some of these big particles including undigested food particles, bad bacteria, and protein like gluten. Among the particles that pass through into your bloodstream are toxic wastes. And because these toxins are foreign substances that are not supposed to be in the bloodstream, this often leads to allergies because the immune system is forced to go into attack mode. In other words, a leaky gut is like an umbrella with holes in it.

So, how do you tell if you have a leaky gut? This syndrome leads to inflammation throughout your system. Basically, a leaky gut affects your whole body. One of the sure warnings of a leaky gut is multiple food sensitivities. Partially, fat and digested protein can seep through the lining of your large intestines, making their way into your bloodstream causing allergic responses. These allergic responses may then manifest themselves as weight gain, digestive problems, skin problems such as acne and rosacea, headaches, joint pain, fatigue, thyroid conditions, syndrome X, food sensitivities and even bloating. Leaving the leaky gut unrepaired can lead to more severe conditions like arthritis, depression, chronic fatigue, muscle pain, migraine headaches, anxiety, candida overgrowth, depression, eczema and inflammatory bowel disease. Studies have also linked a leaky gut to autoimmune diseases such as type 1 diabetes. A leaky gut can also cause mal absorption of vital minerals and nutrients including vitamin B12, zinc and iron.

Before we can look at how to treat a leaky gut, let us first understand what could be its cause so that after treatment, you don't fall back into having a leaky gut.

Causes Of A Leaky Gut

There are five main causes of a leaky gut, namely: bacteria imbalance, dysbiosis, toxin overload, chronic stress, and poor dieting. Understanding this causes will make it easier to find the cure to the syndrome by making simple changes here and there while at home.

Poor dieting

Do you know that proteins can sometimes cause havoc on your intestinal lining? Well, let me be clearer here, I am not just talking about any proteins. The proteins I am referring to are the ones found in un-sprouted grains, conventional diary, GMO foods, and sugar. These proteins turn out to be the most common components of foods that end up damaging the lining of the intestines. For instance, un-sprouted grains contain a large amount of nutrient blockers or anti-nutrients called lectins and phytates.

Lectins happen to be good news for the plant. They are proteins that are bound to sugar molecules and that act as a natural defense system for plants, protecting the plants against outside danger like parasites and mold. Now, this is where the bad news come in. Our digestive lining is covered by sugar-containing cells that help break down our food during the digestion process. When in the body, lectins gravitate towards this area and attach themselves there, damaging our gut and causing inflammation.

Lectins are not only found in grains, these proteins are also found in many other foods like soy, spelt rice and wheat. Consuming them in small amounts will cause you no negative impact. It is when you consume them in large amounts that lead to many problems. When you sprout and ferment grains, you reduce the amount of lectins and phytates present, making them easy to digest. GMO's and foods that are hybridized are modified to fight off bugs making them have very high lectin content. Some grains like wheat also contain gluten, which is another contributor to a leaky gut.

Conventional cow's milk contains protein A1 casein that can harm your gut too. The pasteurization process also destroys vital enzymes making sugars like lactose difficult for the stomach to digest. Sugars also wreak havoc on your digestive system. It feeds the growth of yeast, bad bacteria, and candida, which damages your gut further. For instance, bad bacteria create exotoxins that damage healthy cells and actually create holes in your intestinal walls.

In addition, to the above causes of leaky gut, your leaky gut can also be caused by other things described below:

Chronic Stress

The biochemical changes that occur when you are stressed will have a significant and immediate impact on your gut function. The connection between our gut and our psychology is a two-way path. Bacteria present in the digestive stress can read stress in the body and detect the presence of stress hormones. When this happens, the good bacteria suddenly become pathogenic and rapidly multiply and as a result, the inner ecology of the gut is thrown out of balance leading to a leaky gut. In other words, when you are stressed out, the amount of cortisol, a stress hormone is increased and the result is the degradation of the gut by making it leaky.

Dysbiosis

This condition is among the leading causes of leaky gut. Dysbiosis is an imbalance between the harmful and beneficial species of bacteria in your gut. This condition can begin right from the time you are born, because your mother did not have enough good gut bacteria herself. Too much use of prescription drugs, water with fluoride and chlorine and the lack of foods rich in probiotics can contribute to this imbalance of good-bad bacteria contributing to the development of a leaky gut.

Hormone Imbalances

The health of your gut greatly depends on proper levels of your hormones. When progesterone, estrogen, thyroid or testosterone are out of balance, this can contribute to leaky gut development.

Toxins

Our environment is full of toxins, some of which break down the barriers of the immune system like the gut. The industries that process food also use methods and preservatives that can increase the risk of inflammation of the intestines causing leaky gut. Some of these toxic methods include high-heat processing of sugars, adding excess sugar to processed foods, and deamidating wheat to make it soluble in water.

Autoimmune Conditions

The relationship between autoimmune conditions and a leaky gut is an interesting one. This is because a leaky gut can contribute to autoimmune diseases and vice versa.

On one hand, a leaky gut enables particles to enter into the bloodstream. Such particles are then distributed to other parts and your body views them as threats. As such, it signals the cells to fight against the intruders and this leads to an autoimmune condition.

On the other hand, an autoimmune condition ensures that your body attacks itself. When this happens, your immune system does not discriminate between harmful particles and healthy cells. Thus, it ends up attacking healthy cells and organs, including your gut. This gives birth to a vicious cycle where your leaky gut condition gets worse due to the autoimmune condition.

Of course, other factors can sometimes trigger these conditions including stress or exposure to toxins. In such a situation, the autoimmune condition can contribute to a leaky gut.

Medication

Certain medication like antacids, antibiotics, corticosteroids and some medication for arthritis increase the risk of a leaky gut. Some may be filled with gluten.

Infections

Sometimes ulcers and a leaky gut can be contributed to an overgrowth of a bacterium H.pylori in the stomach. Overgrowth of other harmful bacteria, parasitic infections, intestinal viruses and yeast infection can also cause a leaky gut.

Poor Glutathione Status

Glutathione is our body's primary antioxidant necessary for guarding your cells against damage. It supports the immune function and it is also useful when it comes to detoxifying the body. And when it comes to your gut, glutathione is the one charged with defending and repairing the lining of the gut.

Unfortunately, nowadays, there are a variety of factors that lead to the depletion of glutathione in the human body. Things such as chronic stress, environmental toxins, smoking, poor diet and lifestyle factors deplete the levels of glutathione. When this happens, your body becomes more susceptible to things such as food sensitivities, chronic inflammation, autoimmune diseases and leaky gut.

Next, we will focus on our mucous system.

The Role Of The Mucous System

The mucous system in our nasal passage flashes viral and bacterial particles into our stomach where the hydrochloric acid present in there is supposed to kill them. Any that gets through to a healthy gut is eventually excreted. When you have a leaky gut, this does not happen; rather, it all ends up in your bloodstream. By improving your leaky gut:

You are shielding candida yeast culture roots from leaking into the walls of your intestines hence reducing the chances of development of the disease.

You hinder contaminants that cause allergies such as exhaust gasses, solvents, dust, and pollen from entering the tissues of your lungs and nasal passage thus reducing the effects of asthma and hay fever.

You are shielding parasites such as salmonella, giardia, cryptosporidium from entering the walls of your stomach and intestines and causing diseases.

Toxins and undigested food are stopped from getting into your bloodstream through a gut that is leaky bringing down the common cause of autoimmune disease and allergies.

Let's dive in even further.

The Gut-Brain Axis: How Leaky Gut Leads To Depression, Anxiety And Migraine Headache

The brain and the gut communicate so closely with one another in ways you never imaged. Not only does our gut influence our brain, but also our brain has a great effect on the health of our gut. This is a two-way nature of communication where the communication signals travel from your gut to your brain and back again. Any problem along this path creates a vicious cycle between the two where your gut problems end up triggering neurological symptoms in your brain and this aggravates your gut in return.

Because of this, the gut is sometimes referred to as the 'second brain'. Many of us are affected by this vicious cycle without even knowing it. At some point in our lives, we find ourselves fighting depression, anxiety and migraines and end up treating the symptoms separately often with the use of OCD or/and prescription drugs. We do this without really understanding that whatever we are dealing with is in a way related to our digestion and by simply dealing with the digestion problems, we could relieve ourselves from depression, anxiety and migraines.

14

How Gut-Brain Axis Is Affected By The Leaky Gut

You might be familiar with the expression 'having butterflies in the stomach'. This is common when one is excited, nervous or anxious and it is a way of your body saying that whatever is happening to your mind is not only up there but is also in the gut. There are 3 kinds of messages that are sent through our bodies: neurotransmitters, cytokines and hormones.

When you are unwell or stressed, the first thing that happens is that the bacteria in your gut are thrown out of balance. Secondly, your hormones jump right in and disrupt communication within your digestive system and between your brain and your gut. On the other hand, by eating foods that are sensitive, you trigger cytokine signal molecules that develop due to bacteria imbalance in the intestines and a leaky gut

Once triggered, these messengers travel to your brain from your gut spreading a message of inflammation along the way. The same cytokines from your gut can pass through the blood brain barrier to affect your moods and cause you headaches, otherwise known as the leaky brain.

Neurotransmitters, the third set of messengers are the ones that communicate throughout your nervous system including the one in the digestive system. The vagal nerve is the main communication mechanism in the gut-brain axis. This is an important part of an autonomic nervous system that takes care of other functions such as bowel movement and the heartbeat. The messages of this autopilot system is also carried by the vagal nerve from your brain to your gut as well as from your gut to your brain. Hormones and cytokines from the gut also use the vagal nerve to transfer their message to the brain.

Clearly, you can see how your mind has a direct effect on your digestion. Simple stress remedies can support and release anti-stress messages, depression, anxiety and headaches and other digestive problems. You can stimulate your vagal nerve system by taking control of your gut-brain axis. When you feel anxious, depressed or you are having a headache, performing these simple exercises, will enable you to stimulate your vagal nerve.

Step 1: Take a deep breath, as deep as you can while counting to 5 and then exhale slowly as you can through your mouth with your lips pursed. Repeat for five to 10 minutes.

Step 2: Take a mouthful of liquid, warm in this case, and hold in your mouth while breathing in through your nose for at least 3 minutes

Step 3: Dip your face, in a bowl of cold water at temperature of approximately 50°F for at least 3 minutes. This includes your eyes too.

You can also control your gut-brain axis by controlling your diet to reduce inflammation. You can easily achieve this by avoiding foods that cause you inflammation and the release of cytokines. This includes refined sugars and high fructose corn syrup and food allergens from dairy proteins.

Healing the gut-brain axis and the leaky gut takes a lot of time and will need a lot of patience. While these steps can be overwhelming and frustrating, this is not a reason to give up. Every person is unique in one way or the other so it is not definite how long before you see any improvement. The great thing about healing your gut is that you heal your brain too.

Healing Your Leaky Gut

A leaky gut can be healed with six simple steps. Here are five R's in details explaining how you can heal your gut.

Remove

When dealing with a leaky gut, the first step is to identify the cause of your irritation of the lining of the gut and removing it, rather than using drugs to suppress its symptoms. Some main sources of irritation include:

Gluten

This is a protein that is found in various grains such as rye, barley, wheat, kamut and oats. Various products such as sauces, condiments, packaged food and processed foods often contain gluten.

Here's the thing. Gluten is not something many people tolerate. When they eat it, their stomachs feel bloated, they produce gas and they suffer from an upset stomach. But that's not the only reason to avoid gluten. The truth is that gluten triggers your body's production of zonulin. This protein, when overproduced, causes the junctions of your digestive track to break apart and this leads to a leaky gut.

18

Thus, in order to heal your gut, you'd do well to give it a break to gluten because foods containing gluten damage your gut.

Grains

It is true that not all grains contain gluten. But there is a good reason to avoid grains such as brown rice when you are in the process of treating your gut. Such grains can still damage your gastrointestinal tract. This is because they contain phytic acid. This is a protective coating that is difficult to digest. The bad news is that when food is not digested properly, it often causes intestinal inflammation. In turn, intestinal inflammation makes your job of healing your gut harder.

If you want to eat grains, stick to eating quinoa. This is because it is more of a seed. Remember, the idea is to give your gut room to heal. As such, even if you consider some grains healthy, eating them will not benefit you at this point in your gut healing process.

Refined Sugars

Refined sugars are not good for your gut. Brown sugar, table sugar and high fructose corn syrup contribute to leaky gut simply because they are pro-inflammatory in nature. Such sugars can damage your intestinal lining and as such, contribute to the issue instead of helping alleviate it.

But there is something else.

Processed sugars are basically food for yeast and bacteria that live within your gastrointestinal tract. They contribute to an overgrowth of such bacteria and when that occurs, the bacteria are referred to as bad bacteria due to the fact that they not only outnumber but also deplete the beneficial bacteria. Good or beneficial bacteria are charged with preventing inflammation and keeping your gut clean and healthy. Thus, you can see the importance of preventing the bad bacteria from overgrowing.

When an overgrowth occurs, it is known as gut dysbiosis. This situation contributes to chronic digestive conditions as well as leaky gut. As such, it is not unusual for people who suffer from conditions such as candida to have leaky gut as well. This is why refined sugar should not be in your diet. If you want, you can consume green leaf stevia or low-sugar fruits instead of using refined sugars. But stay away from artificial sweeteners because they may interfere with beneficial gut bacteria.

Refined Vegetables Oils

Refined vegetables oils are obviously bad for you since they have a high omega-6 ratio which is pro-inflammatory especially when consumed in excess. But they are also treated with various chemicals that are bad for the intestinal lining. When trying to heal your gut, you should be careful not to use such oils. Oils such as peanut, canola, sunflower, soybean and safflower oil should not be part of your diet.

All in all, these four foods are the main culprit as far as leaky gut is concerned. You need to eliminate such foods from your diet in order to give your gut room to heal. But apart from doing that, there is something else you should do. You should start an elimination diet to help you pinpoint individual foods that may harm your gut.

Start an elimination diet by removing some common irritants like dairy, soy, gluten, sugar and chemical additives you find in many processed foods. By proper elimination of specific foods in your diet, you can pinpoint which food is exactly causing trouble in your gut. You can do it by eliminating a food or two per week then record all the effects you felt before reintroducing them again. Your gut will tell you what food it is sensitive to; all you have to do is listen. Identifying your problem and removing it from your diet can surprisingly give you quick relief.

Limit your use of NSAIDs and alcohol. Alcohol steals nutrients from your gut besides overworking your liver. NSAIDs are the most common pain relief medicine in the world. In addition to killing pain, NSAIDs lower fever and reduce swelling. The side effect of these drugs is that they inhibit your body's production of prostaglandins, substances you need to rebuild the lining of the intestines. Continuous use of this drug for two weeks puts you at a risk of a leaky gut that will not go away even after you stop the use of the medication.

Root out infections. All the nutrients in the world won't help cure your problems if you have a parasite in your gut. If elimination method fails, then you will have to find a health practitioner for tests and treatment.

Replace

Once you have identified the cause of your gut failure and removed it, the next step would be to give your body what it needs to rebuild the gut lining. You can do this in many different ways, one of them being eating plenty of whole foods. These foods are full of vitamins, enzymes, phytonutrients and minerals your intestines need to heal. Prioritize on lean proteins, healthy fats, and non-starchy vegetables to help strengthen your cellular membrane. Colorful vegetables, nuts and seeds are a good source of fiber. Aim for 30 grams of fiber per day and consider supplementing with 1-2 tablespoons of chia seeds, psyllium seeds, and flaxseed or oat bran.

Also, take digestive enzymes for your intestines. The small intestines has a layer of villi and microvilli projections covered with digestive enzymes that our body needs to break food with during digestion. By supporting these enzymes with supplements, you will be helping rebuild the villi that were damaged. Taking supplemental enzymes before a meal will also give your digestive tract a jump-start on digestion, making food easier to break down and nutrients to assimilate easily. Take a capsule of enzyme supplements with meals three times a day and within a few weeks, your villi will be back on track.

You may also want to supplement with glutamine, an amino acid that will support your digestion and immunity by acting as fuel for the intestinal lining. Also supplement with more omega-3 fatty acids, as your gut will use them to rebuild cell walls that are healthy and calm inflammation. Essential fatty acids will also improve the tight junctions between the gut linings' cells. Take a daily supplement of fish oil supplements or get it directly from omega-3 rich foods including seeds, nuts, avocado and cold-water fish.

Re-Inoculate

Once your body has recovered from the leaks in your gut, it will be great if you help it to grow a layer of good bacteria that will help protect it from future threats while at the same time assist with digestion. These beneficial bacteria will also strengthen your immune system, improve your metabolism, and help your body absorb vitamins and minerals.

You get these bacteria from a probiotic or eating fermented food. High intensity probiotic support revives a micro biome damaged by poor diet or antibiotics. Select a high potency probiotic of many different cultures two times a day. Eating fermented food on the other hand will help to get the probiotic bug to stick around, as well reducing inflammation, improving anti-oxidant status and blood sugar control. You can also get the ingredients necessary to heal your leaky gut from supplements.

Supplements to heal your gut include:

L-Glutamine

L-Glutamine powder is also an essential amino acid supplement that is anti-inflammatory and necessary for the growth and repair of your intestinal lining. L-Glutamine powder acts as a protector coating the wall of your cells and acting as a repellant to irritants. Aim to take 2-5 grams two times a day.

Collagen Protein

Collagen is very important when it comes to healing your gut. This is because it has glycine and poline. These are amino acids that come in handy when repairing damaged cell walls. Collagen protein can be taken as a supplement to help repair the gut lining. It also helps in ensuring you have healthy joints and bones and it is useful in keeping your skin, nails and hair healthy.

GI Repair Powder

GI Repair Powder works to protect intestinal mucosal integrity. It has healing ingredients such as aloe vera, collagen, licorice and L-glutamine that not only heal the gut lining but also ensure that it remains healthy. You'll need to use ½ to 1 teaspoon of the supplement at least 2 to 3 times a day in order to repair your gut lining.

Digestive Enzymes

Digestive enzymes are needed in order to aide digestion. When your body does not have enough of such enzymes, you cannot digest food properly and this poses a risk of leaky gut. Fortunately, you can take digestive enzymes in supplement form. These microbial-based supplements do the important job of supporting the breaking down and absorption of macronutrients. As such, you can take them with your meals to give your body enough enzymes to digest the food you eat properly. This will lessen the strain on your gut and give it time to heal.

Quercetin

Quercetin is something else that can help you heal your gut. This flavonoid works by stabilizing mast cells and thereby reducing the amount of histamine the cells produce. This leads to reduced levels of inflammation and helps guard the gut lining against damage.

Quercetin also does the remarkable job of tightening your intestinal barrier. This helps in re-sealing the leak. As such, you can take 3 to 6 grams of quercetin in powder form daily. This will go a long way in treating your gut.

Vitamins A and D

Vitamins A and D are two vitamins that enable the body to secrete immunoglobulin A. This is a significant ingredient when it comes to enhancing the mucous membranes and boosting the immune system function. When you take vitamin A and D, you be in effect helping to rebuild your gut.

The importance of these supplements is to give you the building blocks to keep your gut healthy. They are just a step in the right direction to healing your gut but you need to take other steps to prevent leaky gut in the future. You need to rebalance your life.

Repair and Rebalance

Once your gut is back on the right track, it is good to think about lifestyle changes that will be lasting. Going back to your old eating habits can easily backtrack all the benefits you gained from healing your gut. Therefore, you would need to make the following changes:

Determine which foods to eat: The best way to keep your gut healthy is by eating foods that will not harm it. Some foods you can eat include:

- **Beverages:** teas, water, bone broth, nut milk, coconut milk, and kombucha

- **Cultured dairy products:** yogurt, Greek yogurt, kefir and traditional buttermilk

- **Fruit:** coconut, grapes, lemon, bananas, raspberries, blueberries, strawberries, oranges, kiwi, pineapple, papaya , mandarin, limes and passion fruit

- **Gluten-free grains:** amaranth, buckwheat, sorghum , gluten-free oats and rice (brown and white)

- **Sprouted seeds:** flax seeds, chia seeds, sunflower seeds, and more

- **Herbs and spices:** all herbs and spices

- **Roots and tubers:** yams, potatoes, squash, sweet potatoes, carrots, , and turnips

- **Fermented vegetables:** tempeh, kimchi, sauerkraut and miso

- **Meats and eggs:** lean cuts of turkey, chicken, lamb, beef and eggs

- **Healthy fats:** coconut oil, avocado, extra virgin olive oil and avocado oil

- **Fish:** herring, salmon, tuna, and other omega-3-rich fish

- **Nuts:** raw nuts, including almonds, peanuts, and nut-based products

- **Vegetables:** broccoli, carrots, Brussels sprouts, arugula, cabbage, kale, eggplant, Swiss chard, beetroot, mushrooms , spinach, ginger and zucchini

The idea is to make a habit of selecting foods that are good for your gut over foods that cause harm to your gut. Remember, it takes time for your gut lining to be damaged. If you keep on eating foods that are bad for your gut, eventually, your gut will pay for it. Thus, try as much as possible to stick to gut healthy foods.

Improve your eating habits: Chew food thoroughly before you swallow to support digestion. Also, visit your dentist frequently to have your teeth checked. Sometimes bacteria from the teeth can spread down your gut, causing multiple other problems like an imbalance in good bacteria that may eventually develop into a leaky gut. Also, do not eat very much when you are stressed or angry. The lining of our stomach produces hydrochloric acid, which produces the correct acidity for digestive enzymes including pepsin. Over the age of 60 years, the deficiency of this acid is a common phenomenon. This acid is also deficient in any person of any age when chronically stressed. This can lead to a weakened digestion and a deficiency of vitamin B 12. This means that you have to increase the content of the acid in the stomach for digestion to take place. One useful technique to do this is to sip on a glass of water containing 2 to 3 tablespoons of good quality organic apple vinegar with juice of half lemon added. You will also find that doing this not only improves digestion but also flatulence and abnormal bloating, all associated with a leaky gut.

Eating mindfully will also save you a lot of trouble: Look at the food before taking the first bite. Pay attention to its flavors and texture while chewing. This will release enzymes by triggering the cephalic phase of digestion that will help in breakdown of food. Take breaths and pauses between bites and avoid multitasking to help your mind focus on digestion.

Relax

One thing you shouldn't neglect in your quest to repair your leaky gut is relaxation. As we've seen, chronic stress can make you susceptible to various conditions including a leaky gut.

As such, you need to research and use various stress management techniques to deal with stressful situations because when you are stressed, your nervous system switches to fight-or-flight mode and the accompanying symptoms that put a toll on your body's immune system.

But the thing with stress is that it can be managed. The first step is to figure out where the stress stems from and decide if it is something that you can avoid. For example, if being around certain people stresses you, you can cut back on the time you spend with them.

If you cannot avoid certain people or situations, you can do other things to alter your situation. For example, you can change how you view a person who stresses you. Instead of being offended, you can learn to take see the meaning behind their actions or you can write them off as people who are ill-mannered and learn to ignore their actions. Alternatively, you can chat with them and tell them how their actions make you feel and work towards a solution.

But even as you strive to free yourself from stress, you have to accept that some things are beyond your control. This will free you as you'll no longer try to control everything. You'll learn to roll with the punches instead of focusing on and stressing over things that you can do nothing about. And above all, you'll find little things that make you happy and include them in your life instead of focusing on the negative things in your life.

The idea is to focus on your happiness, not on the stressful things in life. If you appreciate the good things in life, you'll learn that although stress is real, it does not sum up your life. And if things get too hard, you can also consider daily meditation or practice yoga to help calm your central nervous system.

Home Remedies For Leaky Gut

Severe cases of leaky gut syndrome will have to be treated medically but you can take the initiative to control mild cases with simple home remedies. Below are some of the most effective solutions for a leaky gut and its symptoms when at home.

Peppermint Tea

Peppermint tea soothes the walls of the intestines, promotes the secretion of bile and eradicates bad bacteria and toxins thus preventing them from leaking out into the bloodstream. By getting rid of bad bacteria flourishing in your gut, thanks to its antibiotic property, you lower the probability of infection. In addition to this, peppermint tea also improves digestion. Take two cups of peppermint tea every day to get relief from symptoms of leaky gut.

Chamomile Tea

Drinking 2 cups of chamomile tea per day will provide relief for your stomach. Chamomile tea acts as a natural relaxant. It helps to relieve stress, which is one of the causes of a leaky gut. It also helps to reduce symptoms like stomach pain, flatulence and gives relief to acidity besides relieving stomach cramps caused by a leaky gut.

Ginger

Ginger contains potent healing properties that help to reduce inflammation and irritation caused in the intestinal lining as a result of a leaky gut. That's not all; ginger is rich in different anti-oxidant properties, which are highly potent in helping your body to fight off harmful bacteria, toxins, and microorganisms inside the intestines. This will prevent the pathogens and toxins from finding their way into the bloodstream. Adding more ginger to your daily meals is a considerable effective way of treating the leaky gut syndrome. Drinking ginger tea or chewing ginger, will also give you desirable results.

Garlic

Eating a few cloves of raw garlic everyday can effectively treat a leaky gut. In addition to reducing blood pressure and cholesterol levels in the body, garlic also helps to remove yeast that is in excess from the intestines and stomach. You can also maintain a healthy gut by including garlic in your meals every day as it helps to balance bacteria in the stomach and as a result, treats a leaky gut and prevents cases of reoccurrence. Eating two cloves of garlic, a day can treat the condition.

Water

Consuming an inadequate amount of water can lead to several health ailments including a leaky gut. When you are chronically dehydrated, this can lead to overgrowth of bacteria and inflammation of the bowel lining. Drinking an average of 8 to 10 glasses of water everyday can aid in flushing out the harmful toxins in the intestines, thereby reducing the symptoms of a leaky gut. Less amount of water in your system can lead to chronic dehydration, which would turn cause your bowel content to harden and stagnate regular bowel function, which can lead to bowel disorders. In the long run, this condition leads to a leaky gut. As much as you need drinking water for your system to treat your leaky gut, drinking plain water is the best as compared to beverages like sodas, tea, and sugary drinks as this ends up dehydrating your body and aggravating the symptoms of a condition already existing.

Foods Rich In Fiber

Fiber is very important in enhancing the movement of food through your gut, something that in turn helps prevent instances of blockage that could end up contributing to the development of a leaky gut.

Foods that are high in fiber also tend to be high in different phytonutrients, living enzymes and essential antibiotics that help to fight bad bacteria present in the gut. With the harmful microorganism out of the picture, the gut would have space and time to heal properly. In addition, without fiber, probiotics cannot live. This is why you need a diet rich in fiber like sprouted flaxseed and chia seeds. But if you have a severely leaky gut, you may need to start getting your fiber from steamed fruits and vegetables. The best foods high in fiber are colorful vegetables, seeds, nuts, legumes and whole-kennel grains.

Foods Rich In Probiotics

Consuming foods that are rich in probiotics can greatly help you fight leaky gut along with its symptoms. The term probiotics simply refers to various living microorganisms, which supply the body with lots of good bacteria. The good bacteria can then fight off the bad bacteria inhabiting the stomach intestines. Probiotics also aid in the secretion of inflammatory mediators and development of the immune system. This will promote quick recovery of the condition.

Some of the best natural sources of probiotics include yogurt and other fermented food or supplements.

Echinacea

This herb soothes the epithelial lining of the gastrointestinal system. Echinacea also boosts the immune system so that it is able to fight the toxins better. It is also a good anti-inflammatory herb that prevents inflammation. You can take one ounce of Echinacea extract with ½ cup for water to have the desired effect.

Bone Broth, Coconut And Coconut Products

Bone broth contains collagen. Collagen contains two amino acids; poline and glycine, that help heal the damaged cell walls of the gastrointestinal tract. The gelatin in the bone broth found in feet, knuckles and other joints, help seal up holes in the intestines. This helps cure chronic constipation, diarrhea and even some food intolerance. A cup of bone broth a day will work miracles for your leaky gut syndrome.

Coconut has pro-biotic properties in it that prevents leaky gut condition and makes your digestive system healthy. The MCFA's found in coconut are quite easy to digest when compared to fats from other sources, something that makes them very effective for leaky gut. Also, coconut kefir is rich in probiotics that are very effective in supporting the functioning of your digestive system. Using caprylic acid too, an extract of coconut oil is the solution to the overgrowth of yeast if you are struggling with such. This can help protect you from a leaky gut. This acid is also known for its antiviral and antifungal properties that can heal your gut condition.

Slippery Elm

This miracle herb can cure a leaky gut with just a few days of consumption. Slippery elm is rich in mucilage that can help stimulate the nerve endings and as a result, protect the digestive system. It also has antioxidant properties that can provide relief from the symptoms of a leaky gut.

Carrots

Carrots deserve a special mention in the fight against leaky gut due to their many health benefits. They are packed with Vitamins A, B complex, C, D, E and K and they contain iron, manganese, potassium, iodine, copper, chromium, sulphur, silica and fiber. It's little wonder that carrots are considered as a super vegetable. They not only help metabolism and digestion but also alleviate stomach ulcers and relieve constipation. These are important functions as they promote the health of your gut.

Remember, one reason for leaky gut is food not being digested properly. By aiding digestion and alleviating constipation, carrots give you the tool you need to aide your gut. Another thing carrots do is reduce inflammation. This is another way in which this healthy vegetable helps your gut. You can eat carrots in their raw form, add them in your food or take it in juice form.

Banana

Bananas are good for your gut. They nourish your digestive system and provide your body with calcium, potassium, magnesium and Vitamins B and Vitamin C. They also soothe intestinal inflammation and this helps reduce the risk of leaky gut. You can enjoy eating bananas in their ripe form and you can also add them in smoothies. If you're feeling bloated or your digestive system is irritated, make a banana smoothie by blending together a banana, a pinch of cinnamon and some oat milk. This soothing drink will help you find relief.

Kiwi Fruit

Kiwi fruit is often used as a remedy for constipation. This is because it soothes the gastrointestinal tract. It also happens to be high in soluble fiber. As such, it can be a great help in aiding digestion. In fact, if you eat 2 kiwi fruits each day for a period of one month, you will increase bowel mobility and do away with such things as irritable bowel. You can combine 1 teaspoon of Healthy Chef Greens with a bit of lime juice, water and 2 kiwi fruits. This smoothie will help soothe your gut.

Green Juice

Green juice is often touted as a healthy drink. It has a great dose of living phytonutrients. These phytonutrients happen to be highly alkalizing. This means they can assist you to heal, cleanse and nourish your gut and your body as a whole. This is the main reason green juice is often cited in detox diets. It cleanses the body. It also contains chlorophyll, which acts as a natural deodorizer. This makes it easier to get rid of halitosis and body odor, which are side effects of poor digestion.

Apart from using the various home remedies, something that will really help you repair your leaky gut is embracing dietary changes. Let's look at some recipes you can use to treat leaky gut.

Recipes To Treat Leaky Gut

Drink Recipes

Berry Flax Smoothie

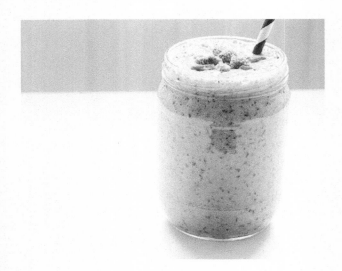

Servings: 1-2

Ingredients

1 teaspoon peeled ginger root

1 tablespoon flax seeds ground

1 cup spinach

½ cup frozen or fresh berries

1 ½ cups dairy free milk

Directions

1. In a high-speed blender, add all the ingredients.

2. Pulse for 2 to 3 minutes or until smooth.

3. Serve.

Healthy Whole Veggie Juice

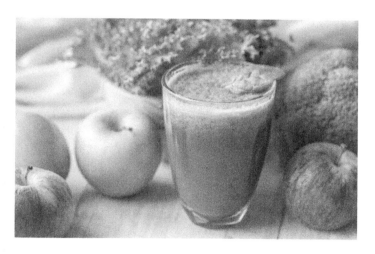

Servings: 4

Ingredients

1/4 teaspoon probiotic powder

2 tablespoons The Myers Way® Collagen Protein (optional)

Herbs of your choice (basil, mint, parsley, cilantro, or fennel)

2 stalks kale

1 inch ginger root

1 lemon

1 green apple

2 cucumbers

Directions

1. Blend the ingredients using a high speed blender.

2. Serve immediately.

Ultimate Gut Health Smoothie

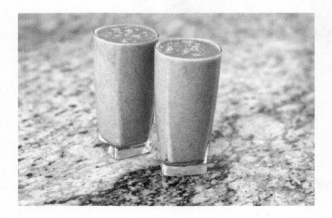

Servings: 1-2

Ingredients

1 ounce aloe vera juice

1 teaspoon vanilla extract

1 teaspoon cinnamon

1 cup spinach or any leafy green

½ cup dairy free kefir or dairy free yogurt unsweetened

½ cup dairy free milk

Directions

1. In a blender, add the ingredients and blend until smooth.

2. Taste and add more vanilla or cinnamon if you wish.

3. Enjoy.

Gut-Healing Smoothie

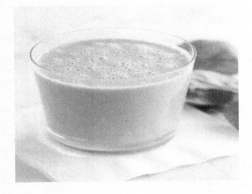

Servings: 4

Ingredients

2 tablespoons The Myers Way® Collagen Protein (optional)

1/4 teaspoon probiotic powder

1/2 cup frozen berry mix (raspberries, strawberries, blueberries)

3 stalks dinosaur kale

3 stalks red kale

3/4 cup unsweetened coconut milk

Directions

1. Add the ingredients into your blender.

2. Blend until smooth.

3. Enjoy.

Chocolate Protein Smoothie

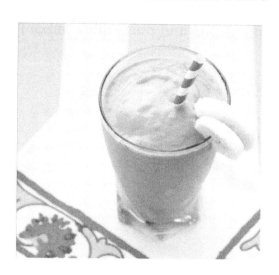

Servings: 1

Honey, optional, to taste

1 teaspoon cinnamon

1 tablespoon carob powder

2 tablespoons collagen (Great Lakes brand)

1 ripe banana

1/4 avocado

1/2 cup coconut milk

1 cup ice

Directions

1. In a blender, add the ingredients and pulse until smooth and creamy.

2. Serve.

Healing Pineapple Smoothie

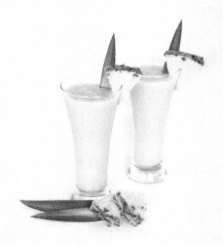

Servings: 2-3

Ingredients

2 inches ginger root

3 inches turmeric root

1 cup young Thai coconut water

2 oranges, squeezed for their juice

1/2 large cucumber

1 small, ripe pineapple, chopped into cubes

Directions

1. Place the ingredients in a powerful blender.

2. Blend for 30 seconds.

3. Serve immediately.

Anti-Inflammatory Turmeric Milk

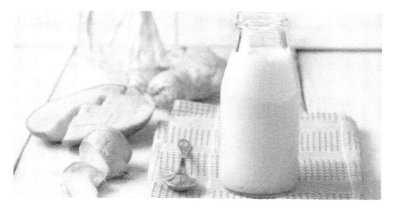

Servings: 2

Ingredients

¼ teaspoon ginger powder

1 teaspoon raw honey

Pinch of black pepper

½ teaspoon cinnamon

2 teaspoons turmeric

2 cups plain coconut milk

Directions

1. Pulse the ingredients in a blender.

2. Once done, place the mixture in a saucepan and proceed to heat over medium heat for 3 to 5 minutes.

3. Serve warm.

Healing Smoothie

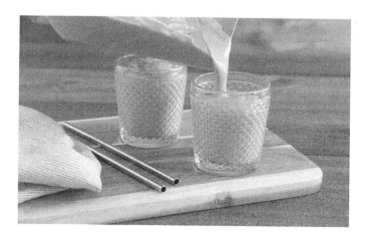

Servings: 4

Ingredients

2 tablespoons collagen protein or whey protein

1 tablespoon raw honey or manuka honey

1 tablespoon hemp hearts

1/2 tablespoon bee pollen

1/2 tablespoon chia or flax seeds

1 teaspoon freshly grated ginger

2 bananas, frozen and cut into chunks

1/2 avocado

2 cups spinach

2 cups kale

1-2 cups full-fat almond milk or coconut milk

Directions

1. Blend the ingredients in a high speed blender for 2 to 3 minutes.

2. Serve over ice.

Gut-Soothing Ginger & Slippery Elm Tea

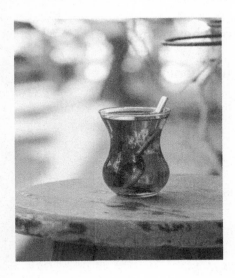

Leaky Gut

Servings: 1 - 2

Ingredients

2 cups purified water

1 teaspoon slippery elm powder

1 teaspoon fresh ginger root

Directions

1. Carefully grate the ginger root and then add it into your teapot.

2. In the teapot, add 2 cups of water and bring the mixture to a boil.

3. Strain the ingredients.

4. Add the slippery elm powder and stir to dissolve.

5. Serve.

53

Aloe Mint Smoothie

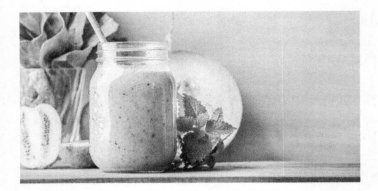

Servings: 1 – 2

Ingredients

3 tablespoon collagen hydrolysate

1/4 inch fresh ginger root

1 sprig fresh mint leaves

1 tablespoon chia or flaxseed

2 tablespoons virgin coconut oil

8 ounces coconut water or filtered water

4 oz. aloe vera juice

1/2 medium avocado

1/2 cup frozen berries

Directions

1. Pulse the ingredients in a blender.

2. Serve.

Breakfast Recipes

Breakfast Bowl With Roasted Strawberries

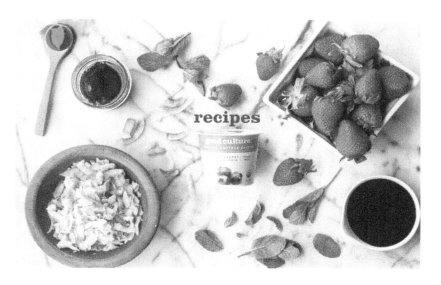

Servings: 2

Ingredients

Fresh mint leaves

2 containers Good Culture blueberry acaí chia cottage cheese

2 tablespoons honey

2 tablespoons balsamic vinegar

8 ounces fresh strawberries, trimmed and halved

Directions

1. Preheat your oven to 375F.

2. In the baking dish, combine the vinegar, honey and strawberry by tossing them together. Roast the ingredients for 30 to 35 minutes or until the strawberries are softened and resemble a syrup,

3. Place a skillet over medium heat. Once done, toast the coconut as you stir frequently. It should be lightly browned and fragrant. Remove and set aside to cool.

4. Add the cottage cheese into a bowl and then add half of the strawberries. Once done, drizzle some balsamic syrup on top.

5. Top with coconut and mint.

6. Enjoy.

Avocado Blueberry Muffins

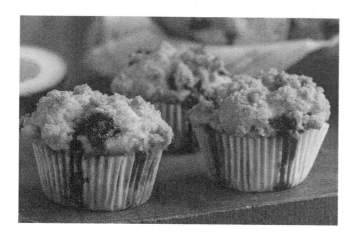

Servings: 12

Ingredients

Muffins:

6 oz. (1 ¼ cup) fresh blueberries

1 cup plain yogurt

1 teaspoon vanilla extract

1 egg

3/4 cup sugar

1 ripe avocado, seeded and peeled

1/2 teaspoon salt

1/2 teaspoon baking soda

2 teaspoons baking powder

2 cups all-purpose flour

Streusel Topping:

1 teaspoon cinnamon

3 tablespoons butter, softened

1/3 cup sugar

1/4 cup flour

Directions

Muffins:

1. Preheat your oven to 375F and then proceed to line the muffin tin using 12 paper liners.

2. In a bowl, combine the baking soda, baking powder, flour and salt.

3. In a stand mixer, add the avocado and beat until it is almost smooth. Add the sugar and continue to beat until well blended. Once done, add the egg and beat to

combine. Add the yogurt and vanilla and make sure you mix well.

4. Sift half of the flour mixture by placing it into a sifter. Add it to the batter in the stand mixer and combine it with the other ingredients.

5. Into the stand mixer, add the remaining flour mixture and combine until just blended.

6. Add the blueberries and fold them into the mixture.

7. Use an ice cream scoop or a spoon to divide the batter equally into the 12 prepared muffin cups.

8. Carefully sprinkle some streusel topping over each cup and then proceed to bake the mixture for 25 to 30 minutes. You can test if it is ready by inserting a wooden tester into the muffins to see if it comes out clean.

9. Allow the muffins to cool on the rack for 5 minutes and then carefully remove them from the cups.

10. Serve warm.

Streusel Topping:

1. Combine the sugar, flour and cinnamon.

2. Add the butter and then proceed to rub it into the dry ingredients by using your fingers. Set aside.

Coconut Chia Pudding

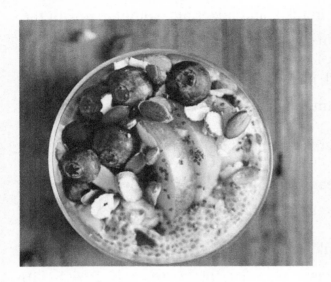

Servings: 4

Ingredients

1 teaspoon cinnamon

2 tablespoons maple syrup

1 tablespoon protein powder of your choice optional

1/4 cup chia seeds (you can use Kunachia brand for extra probiotics)

1 cup coconut milk use the full-fat kind from a can

Directions

1. In a bowl, add all the ingredients and whisk together using a whisk or fork.

2. Cover the mixture and then refrigerate until the pudding is set. You can refrigerate overnight.

3. Top with nuts, fruits and garnishes of your choice.

4. Enjoy.

Matcha And Blueberry Oatmeal

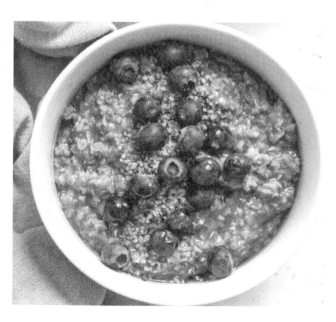

Servings: 2

Ingredients

1 teaspoon vanilla

1/2-1 teaspoon matcha

1 tablespoon chia seeds

2 tablespoons maple syrup

1 scoop Collagen Peptides

1 cup rolled oats

1 1/2 cup almond milk

Toppings

2 tablespoons of hemp seeds

1/2 cup blueberries

Directions

1. In a medium saucepan, mix together the maple syrup, vanilla and almond milk and then bring the mixture to a boil.

2. Add the chia seeds, oats, collagen and matcha and stir to combine.

3. Simmer the ingredients for 3 to 5 minutes. The milk should be absorbed.

4. Divide into individual bowls and then top with hemp seeds and blueberries. Top with some maple syrup on top.

5. Enjoy.

Chocolate Quinoa Breakfast Bowl

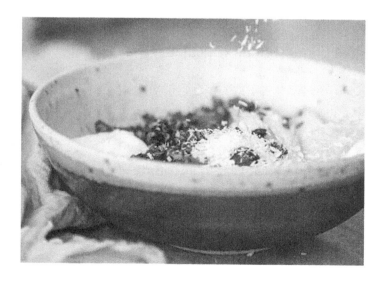

Servings: 2

Ingredients

For the Quinoa Granola

2.5 ounces dark chocolate aim for at least 80% cacao, chopped

2 teaspoons pure maple syrup

2 teaspoons ground flax

1/2 cup mixed seeds and nuts of choice

1 1/2 cups cooked quinoa about 3/4 cup dry

1 tablespoon coconut oil

To assemble

2 teaspoons unsweetened desiccated coconut

1 lime peeled and sliced

1 cup fresh blueberries

1 ripe mango peeled, pitted and sliced

1 cup natural yogurt

Directions

1. Start by heating the coconut oil in a non-stick skillet placed over medium heat. Once the oil is ready, add the quinoa granola ingredients but don't add the chocolate.

2. Stir the ingredients and proceed to cook for 7 to 10 minutes as you stir frequently.

3. Once the time is up, turn off the heat. Add the chocolate and stir.

4. Place the yogurt into individual bowls and then top with the quinoa granola/

5. Serve with coconut flakes and fresh fruit.

Coconut Bircher Muesli

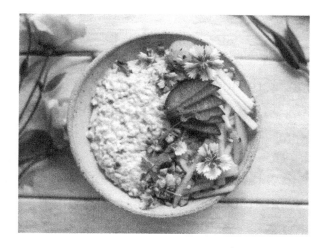

Servings: 1

Ingredients

Seasonal berries to serve

Tahini to serve

2 tablespoons coconut yoghurt

2 tablespoons almonds roughly chopped

1 tablespoon linseeds

1/4 teaspoon vanilla essence or powder

1/4 apple finely julienned (cut into matchsticks)

1/2 cup coconut milk drinking

1/2 cup rolled oats

Directions

1. In a bowl or jar, add all the ingredients minus the coconut yogurt and then mix well. Once done, place the jar in the refrigerator overnight.

2. Once you're ready to eat, add the coconut yogurt and mix and then top with your fruit of choice and a bit of tahini.

3. Enjoy.

Cultured Breakfast Macro Bowls

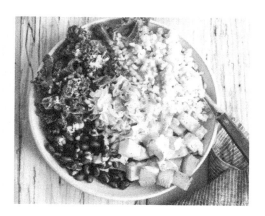

Servings: 4

Ingredients

Sesame seeds, gomasio or chopped green onion, for topping (optional)

Yum sauce for drizzling (optional)

1 cup of kimchi or Farmhouse Culture Kraut

1 ½ cups of black beans (cooked)

1 can beans, drained and rinsed

1 small (chopped) bunch of curly or dinosaur kale stems

Coarse salt and freshly ground black pepper

2 tablespoons vegetable oil such as safflower or grapeseed

6 large or 8 small scrubbed or peeled carrots

2 small or 1 large scrubbed or peeled turnip

2 small or 1 large scrubbed or peeled rutabaga

1 cup short-grain brown rice

Directions

1. Preheat the oven to 425F.

2. In the meantime, cook the rice as per the instructions on the package.

3. Use some to toss the root vegetables and then place the vegetables on a baking sheet lined with foil. Season with pepper and sea salt and then proceed to roast the ingredients for 35 to 40 minutes. The vegetables should be tender. Make sure you stir the vegetables halfway through cooking.

4. Boil some water in a pot and then place a steamer attachment inside and proceed to steam the kale until it is bright green and tender. This should take 3 minutes.

5. Divide the kale, black beans, roasted vegetables and cooked rice into four bowls. Once done, top each bowl with the fermented vegetables and then with some yum sauce or toppings of choice.

6. Serve and enjoy.

Lunch Recipes

Easy Sauerkraut Salad

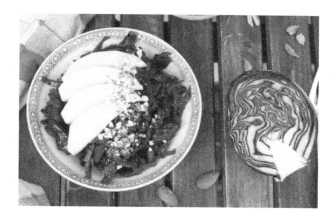

Servings: 2

Ingredients

Freshly ground black pepper

Salt

A dash of chili powder

1 teaspoon minced ginger

1 teaspoon brown sugar

1 teaspoon Dijon mustard

1 tablespoon apple cider vinegar

Seeds of 3-4 green cardamom pods ground

Zest and juice of 1/2 lemon

3 tablespoons extra virgin olive oil

For the salad:

4 tablespoons ground almonds

1/2 ripe mango

200 grams or 7 oz Russian-style sauerkraut

Directions

1. Prepare the dressing: In a bowl, mix together the lemon juice, lemon zest, extra virgin olive oil, Dijon mustard, ground cardamom seeds, minced ginger, freshly ground black pepper, apple cider vinegar, brown sugar and a pinch of salt.

2. Assemble the salad: In a medium sized bowl, add the sauerkraut and then add the dressing and stir to combine.

3. Divide the sauerkraut into individual bowls and then proceed to peel the mango. Add it on top of each bowl and then add the ground almonds.

4. Serve and enjoy.

Bulgogi Tofu Bowls With Kimchi

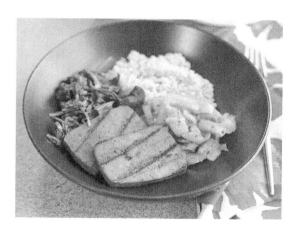

Servings: 2

Ingredients

For bulgogi tofu:

Oil for grill grate if necessary

1/2 cup kimchi drained

10 ounces super firm tofu in vacuum packaging cut in 1/2 inch slices

Grind black pepper

3 garlic cloves minced

1/2 teaspoon ginger powder

1 teaspoon granulated onion

1/4 teaspoon toasted sesame oil

1 teaspoon brown rice vinegar

1 Tablespoon agave syrup

1 Tablespoon gochujang

1/4 cup tamari

For bowls:

1 cup cooked brown rice

Salt to taste

6 ounces baby spinach leaves

2 cloves garlic minced

1/2 teaspoon extra virgin olive oil

Directions

1. To make the bulgogi tofu: Start by adding the agave syrup, ground black pepper, granulated onion, toasted sesame oil, ginger powder, minced garlic, gochujang, tamari, vinegar and brown rice.

2. Once done, add the tofu slices in the marinade. Flip the slices to coat both sides and then allow them to marinate for at least 8 hours. You can marinate for up to 24 hours if you wish. Flip halfway through as you marinate.

3. Once the tofu is done marinating, heat an outdoor grill to 500 degrees. You can lightly oil the grill grate if need be. Proceed to grill the tofu slices for 2 to 3 minutes per side or until you see brown grill marks. Set aside.

4. To make the bowls: Place a non-stick skillet over medium heat. Once done, add some extra virgin olive oil and then proceed to sauté the garlic until fragrant. Add the baby spinach and stir until just wilted. Season with salt.

5. Place a half cup of rice into each bowl. Once done, add the sautéed spinach in thebowls and then top with kimchi and 2 slices of tofu.

6. Serve and enjoy.

Pan-Seared Lemon Turmeric Chicken Salad

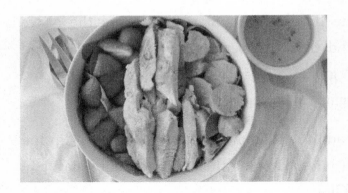

Servings: 2

Ingredients

For the salad:

6 cups fresh spinach

1 cup strawberries

1 tablespoon olive oil

Zest of 1 lemon, plus a drizzle of lemon juice

1 teaspoon turmeric

1 teaspoon sea salt

1 lb. chicken breast

1 medium sweet potato

For the dressing:

1/8 teaspoon freshly cracked black pepper

1/4 teaspoon sea salt

Juice of 1 lemon

¼ cup olive oil

Directions

1. If you don't have a roasted sweet potato, you can roast one for one hour at 350F. You should peel it and slice it into rounds.

2. In the meantime, place a large skillet over medium heat. Use turmeric, 1 teaspoon of sea salt, lemon juice and lemon zest to season the chicken all round. Once the skillet is ready, add 1 tablespoon of olive oil and then cook the chicken for 10 minutes before flipping and cooking for 10 minutes more. Slice the chicken into strips.

3. Carefully slice the strawberries.

4. In a large salad bowl, add the spinach and then add the chicken, sweet potato and strawberries.

5. Prepare the dressing: In a bowl, combine the lemon juice, ¼ cup of olive oil, black pepper and ¼ teaspoon of sea salt.

6. Drizzle the dressing over the salad.

7. Serve.

Basic Broiled Salmon

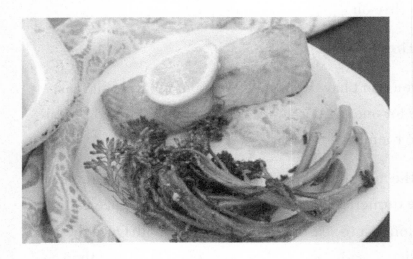

Servings: 2

Ingredients

1–2 lemons, sliced

2 tablespoons sea salt

2 tablespoons olive oil

4 salmon fillets

Directions

1. Turn your broiler on high and then lightly grease a tray or pan. Alternatively, you can line it with parchment paper.

2. Gently pat dry the salmon fillets. Once done, rub them with salt and olive oil.

3. Place the fillets on the top rack in the oven and cook for 10 minutes per inch of thickness.

4. Once done, garnish with lemon slices and serve.

Broccoli Cauliflower Soup

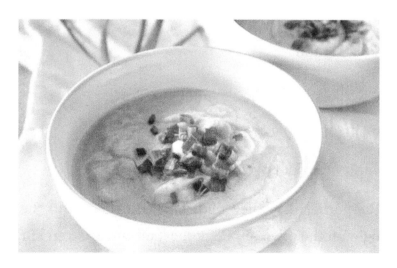

Servings: 2

Ingredients

Optional: black pepper, extra sea salt, extra olive oil and 2 chives

2 teaspoons sea salt

1/2 cup coconut milk

1 cup bone broth

2 cups cauliflower florets

2 cups broccoli florets

1 garlic clove

1/2 yellow diced onion

2 tablespoons olive oil

Directions

1. Place a large stock pot over medium-low heat.

2. Mince the garlic, slice the onion and add them into the pot along with the olive oil. Cook for 5 minutes as you stir occasionally. The onions should be translucent.

3. Add the cauliflower, broccoli, coconut milk, sea salt and bone broth. Set the heat to medium-high and allow the vegetables to cook until they are fork tender.

4. Transfer the ingredients to a blender and pulse until well combined. Alternatively, you can use an immersion blender to create the soup.

5. Sprinkle the chopped chives on top and then add some olive oil and sea salt to taste.

6. Serve.

Grilled Chicken Thighs

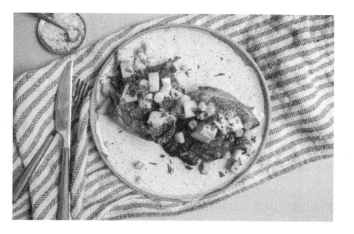

Servings: 6

Ingredients

For the chicken:

3 lbs. bone-in, skin-on chicken thighs

½ teaspoon garlic powder

½ teaspoon ginger powder

½ teaspoon sea salt

For the salsa:

½ lemon, juiced

½ teaspoon ginger powder

½ teaspoon sea salt

1 clove garlic, minced

1 oz. fresh mint leaves, finely chopped

1 bunch green onions, root and top ends removed and finely chopped

1 avocado, chopped

1 medium cucumber, chopped

1 bunch radishes with the tops removed and chopped

½ large pineapple, chopped

Directions

1. Preheat the grill.

2. In a small bowl, combine the spices and salt and set aside.

3. Use a piece of paper towel to dry the chicken well. Set aside as the grill warms up.

4. Before cooking the chicken, use your fingers to rub it well with the spice mixture.

5. Once the grill is hot, carefully arrange the chicken on it with the skin-side down. Cook the chicken for 5 to 7 minutes and then flip it and cook for 5 to 7 minutes more. The thermometer should read 165F.

6. In a bowl, combine the salsa ingredients.

7. Serve the chicken with the salsa.

8. Enjoy.

Pumpkin Curry With Chickpeas

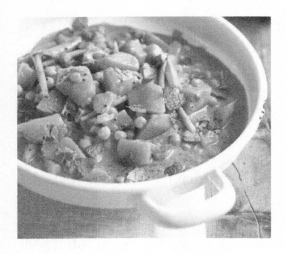

Servings: 4

Ingredients

Naan bread, to serve

Large handful mint leaves

2 limes

400g can chickpea, drained and rinsed

400ml can reduced-fat coconut milk

250ml vegetable stock

1 piece pumpkin or a small squash (about 1kg)

1 tablespoon mustard seed

6 cardamom pods

3 large stalks lemongrass, bashed with the back of a knife

2 onions, finely chopped

3 tablespoons Thai yellow curry paste, or vegetarian alternative

1 tablespoon sunflower oil

Directions

1. Start by heating the oil in a sauté pan and then add some onions, cardamom, lemongrass and mustard seeds and then fry the curry paste for 2 to 3 minutes.

2. Add the squash or pumpkin and stir well to coat with the paste.

3. Add the coconut milk and stock and then allow the ingredients to come to a simmer.

4. Add the chickpeas and cook for 10 minutes. The pumpkin should be tender. If you want to freeze the curry, you can cool it at this stage and freeze it for up to a month.

5. Add the juice of one lime into the curry. Slice the other lime into wedges.

6. Serve curry over mint leaves with lime wedges and warm naan bread.

Dinner Recipes

Roasted Baby Carrot Salad With Walnuts

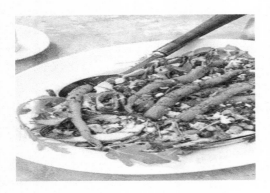

Servings: 4

Ingredients

Seeds from half a pomegranate

100g feta, crumbled

Small bunch coriander, chopped

30g walnut pieces, gently toasted in a dry pan

1 large bag of rocket

100g ready cooked or canned Puy lentils

1 small avocado, sliced

2 tablespoons olive oil

1 teaspoon ground cumin

1 red onion, roughly chopped

Bunch of about 12 young slim carrots, leaves and ends trimmed

For the dressing:

Squeeze of lemon

2 tablespoons virgin olive oil

1 clove garlic, crushed (optional)

2 tablespoons pomegranate molasses

Directions

1.   Preheat your oven to 200 degrees C.

2. Wash the carrots well and leave them unpeeled. Arrange them in a roasting tray. Add the red onion, ground cumin and then some olive oil.

3. Cook the onions and carrots in the oven for 20 to 30 minutes. They should be tender. Once done, remove them from the oven and let them cool slightly.

4. In a jar, add the dressing ingredients and then proceed to shake well in order to combine everything. Taste and adjust the seasoning as necessary.

5. In a bowl, combine the rest of the salad ingredients, half of the dressing and the cooked carrots.

6. Drizzle the remaining dressing on top and serve.

Oriental Tofu Rice Noodles

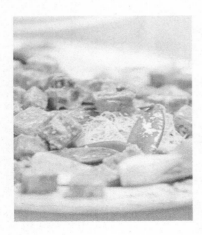

Servings: 4

Ingredients

Salt to taste

1-2 red chillis, depending on preference

1-2 tablespoons chilli infused olive oil

400g cauldron original tofu, cubed

Juice and zest of 1 lime

6 tablespoons almond nut butter

20 pods mangetout

4 pak choy

1 teaspoon each of turmeric powder that has been mixed with peanut butter well and cumin powder

Rice noodles

Directions

1. Boil 100ml of water and then add in the lime juice, zest and almond nut butter and mix well. Once the mixture cools, add the drained tofu. Make sure you coat it well and

then let it rest for at least 30 minutes. You can refrigerate it overnight if you wish.

2. Prepare the noodles according to the instructions on the package and then drain and set aside.

3. In the meantime, proceed to stir fry the mangetout in olive oil infused with chilli. Add the pak choy and cook for 2 minutes more or until softened.

4. Add the tofu, the marinade and the drained noodles. Cook until just heated through.

5. Remove and serve.

Thai Coconut Turkey Soup

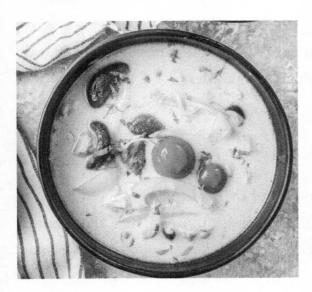

Leaky Gut

Servings: 6

Ingredients

Cilantro, to garnish

Salt to taste

Juice from 1 lime, about 2 tablespoons

3 cups of bean sprouts

1 pint of cherry tomatoes

2 yellow bell peppers, thinly sliced

2 tablespoons coco aminos (can substitute soy sauce)

3 tablespoons green Thai curry paste

1 15-ounce can coconut milk

2 cups shredded cooked turkey meat

8 cups homemade turkey stock

1-inch piece of ginger, julienned

3 garlic cloves, finely minced

5 ounces shiitake mushrooms, cut in half

½ medium onion, thinly sliced

1 tablespoon coconut oil

Directions

1. In a large pot placed over medium-high heat, heat the oil and then add the onion. Cook the onion for 3 minutes or until softened.

2. Add the mushrooms and proceed to cook for 5 minutes.

3. Add the ginger and garlic and cook for 1 minute.

4. Add the shredded turkey, curry paste, coco aminos, coconut milk and turkey stock. Bring the ingredients to a boil. Once done, reduce the heat and then simmer the ingredients for 5 minutes.

5. Add the cherry tomatoes and the bell peppers. Cook for 1 minute.

6. Turn off the heat and then add the lime juice and the bean sprout.

7. Season with salt and garnish with cilantro.

8. Serve.

Spicy Avocado Shrimp Tower

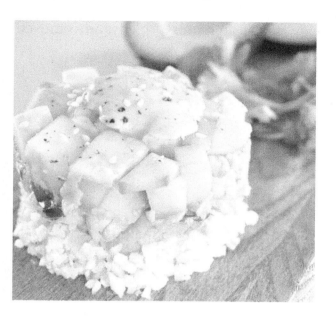

Servings: 4

Ingredients

Black pepper to taste

1 tablespoon sesame seeds

1/3 cup Paleo mayonnaise

2 teaspoon Sriracha sauce

1 tablespoon Coconut Aminos

1 tablespoon sesame oil

1 tablespoon cilantro (finely chopped)

1 cup cooked shrimp (with their tails peeled and removed and then chopped coarsely)

1 cup cucumber (peeled and diced)

1 cup avocado (diced)

1 cup cauliflower rice

Directions

1. In a food processor, pulse the cauliflower into cauliflower rice - they should be finely chopped.

2. In a bowl, combine the sesame oil and cauliflower rice. Set aside.

3. In a small bowl, mash the avocado. It should be slightly chunky. Once done, stir in the cilantro.

4. In another bowl, combine the shrimp and coconut aminos.

5. Mix together the mayonnaise and sriracha sauce.

6. In a cup, add ¼ cup of cucumber, then add the avocado and shrimp and top with cauliflower rice. Press the

ingredients into the cup before flipping the cup onto a plate.

7. Top with mayo, black pepper and sesame seeds.

8. Enjoy.

Dill And Bean Pilaf With Garlicky Yogurt

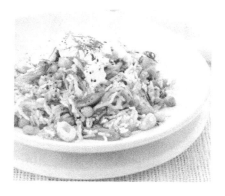

Servings: 2

Ingredients

½ garlic clove, crushed

1 tablespoon milk

100g Greek yogurt

300g of frozen mixed vegetables (containing green beans, peas and, broad beans)

500ml vegetable stock

20g pack dill with the fronds and stalks chopped but kept separate

175g basmati rice

25g butter

2 onions halved and thinly sliced

Directions

1. In a pan, add the butter and fry the onions. Add the dill stalks and rice and stir.

2. Add the saffron stock and bring the ingredients to a boil. Once done, cover the pan and simmer the ingredients for 5 minutes.

3. Add half the dill and the beans and cook for 5 minutes more. The liquid should be absorbed into the rice.

4. In the meantime, combine the garlic, milk, seasoning and yogurt.

5. Pour the mixture on top of the rice and then spread the remaining dill on top.

6. Serve.

Exotic Avocado Salad

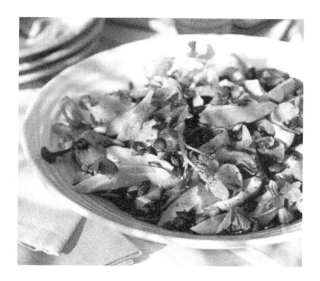

Servings: 2

Ingredients

1 tablespoon olive oil

Juice of 1/2 lime

1/2 small pack fresh mint

50g bag trimmed and washed watercress

1 ripe avocado

1 ripe papaya

2 tablespoons pumpkin seeds

Directions

1. In a frying pan, add the pumpkin seeds and stir until toasted. Remove and allow them to cool.

2. Peel the papayas, scoop out the seeds and slice the papaya thinly. Slice the avocado into half and remove the seed and skin before slicing it thinly.

3. In a large bowl, add the sliced avocados, papayas and pumpkin seeds.

4. Chop the mint and proceed to season with some salt and pepper. Pour the mixture over the salad in the large bowl and use your hands to mix the ingredients.

5. Serve.

Lentils With Homemade Pork

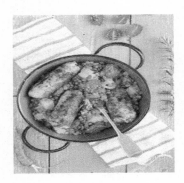

Servings: 4

Ingredients

240g canned green lentils, drained

10 cherry tomatoes

100g celeriac, finely diced

150g potato, finely diced

1 carrot, finely diced

3 tablespoons olive oil

Salt and black pepper

1 teaspoon chopped rosemary

1 teaspoon fennel seeds

2 tablespoons dry white wine

500g minced pork

Directions

1. Combine the pork, fennel seeds, rosemary, wine, salt and pepper. Once done, divide the mixed ingredients into 8

and proceed to form each portion into an 8cm sausage shape. The sausages should be about 3cm in diameter.

2. Wrap the sausages tightly in a piece of foil. Carefully twist the ends of the foil.

3. Place water in a large pan and bring it to a boil. Once done, add the wrapped sausages and cook for 3 minutes. This will allow the sausages to stick together. Once done, let them cool before removing the foil.

4. In a frying pan, add 2 tablespoons of oil and proceed to brown the sausages.

5. In a pan, add 1 tablespoon of oil. add the carrots, celeriac and potatoes and stir,

6. Add a bit of water and then add the cherry tomatoes and cover the pan with a lid. Cook for 5 minutes. The vegetables should be soft.

7. Add the lentils and then arrange the sausages on top.

8. Simmer for 5 minutes.

9. Serve while hot.

4 Weeks Meal Plan

Week One

Day 1

Breakfast: Berry flax smoothie

Lunch: Pan-seared lemon turmeric chicken salad

Dinner: Exotic avocado salad

Day 2

Breakfast: Breakfast bowl with roasted strawberries

Lunch: Broccoli cauliflower soup

Dinner: Lentils with homemade pork

Day 3

Breakfast: Healthy whole veggie juice

Lunch: Grilled chicken thighs

Dinner: Bean & dill pilaf with garlicky yogurt

Day 4

Breakfast: Coconut chia pudding

Lunch: Pumpkin curry with chickpeas

Dinner: Oriental tofu rice noodles

Day 5

Breakfast: Ultimate gut health smoothie

Lunch: Bulgogi tofu bowls with kimchi

Dinner: Thai coconut turkey soup

Day 6

Breakfast: Chocolate quinoa breakfast bowl

Lunch: Easy sauerkraut salad

Dinner: Spicy avocado shrimp tower

Day 7

Breakfast: Gut healing smoothie

Lunch: Basic broiled salmon

Dinner: Roasted baby carrot salad with walnuts

Week Two

Day 1

Breakfast: Chocolate protein smoothie

Lunch: Bulgogi tofu bowls with kimchi

Dinner: Exotic avocado salad

Day 2

Breakfast: Avocado blueberry muffins

Lunch: Easy sauerkraut salad

Dinner: Lentils with homemade pork

Day 3

Breakfast: Healing pineapple smoothie

Lunch: Pan-seared lemon turmeric chicken salad

Dinner: Bean & dill pilaf with garlicky yogurt

Day 4

Breakfast: Matcha and blueberry oatmeal

Lunch: Pumpkin curry with chickpeas

Dinner: Spicy avocado shrimp tower

Day 5

Breakfast: Anti-inflammatory turmeric milk

Lunch: Basic broiled salmon

Dinner: Thai coconut turkey soup

Day 6

Breakfast: Healing smoothie

Lunch: Broccoli cauliflower soup

Dinner: Oriental tofu rice noodles

Day 7

Breakfast: Coconut bircher muesli

Lunch: Grilled chicken thighs

Dinner: Roasted baby carrot salad with walnuts

Week Three

Day 1

Breakfast: Gut-soothing ginger & slippery elm tea

Lunch: Easy sauerkraut salad

Dinner: Lentils with homemade pork

Day 2

Breakfast: Aloe mint smoothie

Lunch: Bulgogi tofu bowls with kimchi

Dinner: Exotic avocado salad

Day 3

Breakfast: Cultured breakfast macro bowls

Lunch: Broccoli cauliflower soup

Dinner: Bean & dill pilaf with garlicky yogurt

Day 4

Breakfast: Berry flax smoothie

Lunch: Pumpkin curry with chickpeas

Dinner: Spicy avocado shrimp tower

Day 5

Breakfast: Breakfast bowl with roasted strawberries

Lunch: Grilled chicken thighs

Dinner: Thai coconut turkey soup

Day 6

Breakfast: Healthy whole veggie juice

Lunch: Basic broiled salmon

Dinner: Oriental tofu rice noodles

Day 7

Breakfast: Coconut chia pudding

Lunch: Pan-seared lemon turmeric chicken salad

Dinner: Roasted baby carrot salad with walnuts

Week Four

Day 1

Breakfast: Ultimate gut health smoothie

Lunch: Easy sauerkraut salad

Dinner: Lentils with homemade pork

Day 2

Breakfast: Chocolate quinoa breakfast bowl

Lunch: Pumpkin curry with chickpeas

Dinner: Exotic avocado salad

Day 3

Breakfast: Gut healing smoothie

Lunch: Broccoli cauliflower soup

Dinner: Bean & dill pilaf with garlicky yogurt

Day 4

Breakfast: Chocolate protein smoothie

Lunch: Grilled chicken thighs

Dinner: Spicy avocado shrimp tower

Day 5

Breakfast: Avocado blueberry muffins

Lunch: Pan-seared lemon turmeric chicken salad

Dinner: Thai coconut turkey soup

Day 6

Breakfast: Healing pineapple smoothie

Lunch: Bulgogi tofu bowls with kimchi

Dinner: Oriental tofu rice noodles

Day 7

Breakfast: Matcha and blueberry oatmeal

Lunch: Basic broiled salmon

Dinner: Roasted baby carrot salad with walnuts

Conclusion

Home remedies are a great step towards curing your leaky gut without really having to go to the doctor but if symptoms persist, you have no other option than visiting a medical practitioner for further diagnosis and treatment.

Made in the USA
Monee, IL
03 December 2020